Delicious Diabetic Pressure Pot Recipes

50 Delicious Diabetic Pressure Pot Recipes for Tasty and Healthy Meals

Cassandra Lane

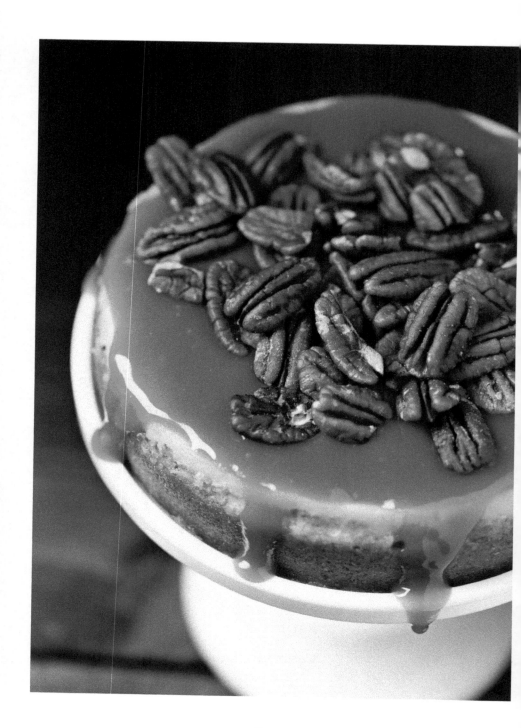

By reading this document, the reader agrees that under no circumstances is the author responsible for any losses, direct or indirect, which are incurred as a result of the use of information contained within this document, including, but not limited to, — errors, omissions, or inaccuracies.

Table of Contents

Korean-Inspired Beef

Servings: 6

Cooking Time: 10 Minutes

Ingredients:

- ¼ cup low-sodium beef broth or Vegetable Broth
- ¼ cup low-sodium gluten-free tamari or soy sauce
- 2 tablespoons rice wine vinegar
- 2 teaspoons Sriracha sauce (optional)
- 2 tablespoons brown sugar
- 1 tablespoon sesame oil
- 3 tablespoons minced garlic
- 1 tablespoon peeled and minced fresh ginger
- ½ teaspoon onion powder
- 1 teaspoon freshly ground black pepper
- 2 pounds top round beef, cut into thin, 3-inch-long strips
- 2 tablespoons cornstarch
- 1 teaspoon sesame seeds
- 2 scallions, green parts only, thinly sliced

Directions:

1. in a 2-cup measuring cup or medium bowl, whisk together the broth, tamari, vinegar,

Sriracha (if using), brown sugar, sesame oil, garlic, ginger, onion powder, and pepper.

2. in the electric pressure cooker, combine the beef and broth mixture; stir.

3. Close and lock the lid of the pressure cooker. Set the valve to sealing.

4. Cook on high pressure for 10 minutes.

5. When the cooking is complete, hit Cancel and quick release the pressure.

6. Once the pin drops, unlock and remove the lid.

7. Using a slotted spoon, transfer the beef to a serving bowl. Hit Sauté/More.

8. in a small bowl, combine the cornstarch and 3 tablespoons of cold water to make a slurry. Whisk the cornstarch mixture into the liquid in the pot and cook, stirring frequently, for about 2 minutes or until the sauce has thickened. Hit Cancel.

9. Pour the sauce over the beef and garnish with the sesame seeds and scallions.

10. Nutrition info: Per serving: Calories: 328; Total Fat: 15g; Protein: 35g; Carbohydrates: 13g; Sugars: 4g; Fiber: 2g; Sodium: 490mg

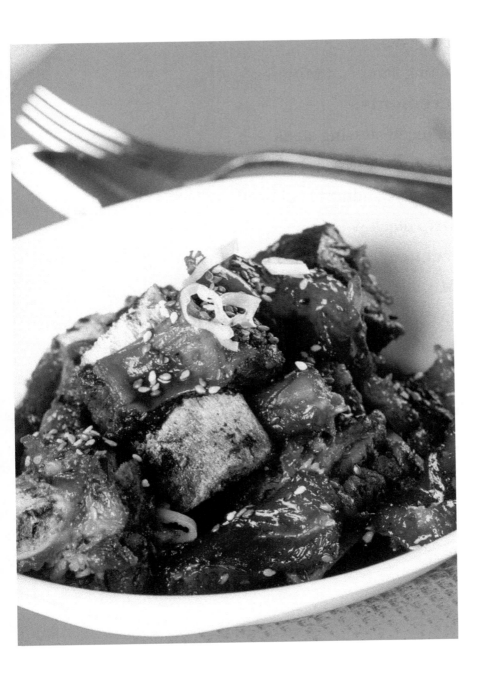

Traditional Beef Stew

Servings: 2

Cooking Time: 35 Minutes

Ingredients:

- 1lb diced stewing steak
- 1lb chopped vegetables
- 1 cup low sodium beef broth
- 1tbsp black pepper

Directions:

1. Mix all the ingredients in your Pressure Pot.

2. Cook on Stew for 35 minutes. Release the pressure naturally.

3. Nutrition info: Per serving: Calories: 0;Carbs: 6 ;Sugar: 1 ;Fat: 9 ;Protein: 43 ;GL: 2

Honey Mustard Pork

Servings: 2

Cooking Time: 60 Minutes

Ingredients:

• 1.5lb rolled, trimmed pork joint

• 1 cup honey mustard sauce, low carb

• salt and pepper

Directions:

1. Mix all the ingredients in your Pressure Pot.

2. Cook on Stew for 60 minutes.

3. Release the pressure naturally.

4. Nutrition info: Per serving: Calories: 290;Carbs: 9 ;Sugar: 8 ;Fat: 17 ;Protein: 39 ;GL: 4

5-Ingredient Mexican Lasagna

Servings: 4

Cooking Time: 15 Minutes

Ingredients:

• Nonstick cooking spray

• ½ (15-ounce) can light red kidney beans, rinsed and drained

• 4 (6-inch) gluten-free corn tortillas

• 1½ cups cooked shredded beef, pork, or chicken

• 1⅓ cups salsa

• 1⅓ cups shredded Mexican cheese blend

Directions:

1. Spray a 6-inch springform pan with nonstick spray. Wrap the bottom in foil.

2. in a medium bowl, mash the beans with a fork.

3. Place 1 tortilla in the bottom of the pan. Add about ⅓ of the beans, ½ cup of meat, ⅓ cup of salsa and ⅓ cup of cheese. Press down. Repeat for 2 more layers. Add the remaining tortilla and press down. Top with the remaining salsa and cheese. There are no beans or meat on the top layer.

4. Tear off a piece of foil big enough to cover the pan

and spray it with nonstick spray. Line the pan with the foil, sprayed side down.

5. Pour 1 cup of water into the electric pressure cooker.

6. Place the pan on the wire rack and carefully lower it into the pot. Close and lock the lid of the pressure cooker. Set the valve to sealing.

7. Cook on high pressure for 15 minutes.

8. When the cooking is complete, hit Cancel. Allow the pressure to release naturally for 10 minutes, then quick release any remaining pressure.

9. Once the pin drops, unlock and remove the lid.

10. Using the handles of the wire rack, carefully remove the pan from the pot. Let the lasagna sit for 5 minutes. Carefully remove the ring.

11. Slice into quarters and serve.

12. Nutrition info: Per serving: Calories: 395; Total Fat: 16g; Protein: 30g; Carbohydrates: 34g; Sugars: 5g; Fiber: 9g; Sodium: 1140mg

Lamb Steaks

Servings: 4

Cooking Time: 50 Minutes

Ingredients:

- 1½ pound lamb steak
- 1 medium white onion, peeled and minced
- 2 teaspoons minced garlic
- 1 teaspoon grated ginger
- 1 ½ teaspoon salt
- 1 tablespoon sugar
- 1 teaspoon ground black pepper
- 3 tablespoons sesame oil
- ¼ cup soy sauce
- 2 tablespoons lemon juice
- 1 cup water
- 1 tablespoon corn starch

Directions:

1. Plugin Pressure Pot, insert the inner pot, press sauté/simmer button, add oil and when hot, add lamb steak and cook for 3 minutes per side or until nicely browned.

2. Add onion, garlic, and ginger and continue cooking

for minutes.

3. Add remaining ingredients except for cornstarch, then press the cancel button, shut the Pressure Pot with its lid and turn the pressure knob to seal the pot.

4. Press the „manual" button, then press the „timer" to set the cooking time to 30 minutes and cook at high pressure, Pressure Pot will take 5 minutes or more for building its inner pressure.

5. When the timer beeps, press „cancel" button and do natural pressure release for 10 minutes and then do quick pressure release until pressure nob drops down.

6. Open the Pressure Pot, transfer lamb steaks to a plate and keep warm.

7. Press the sauté/simmer button, stir cornstarch into the cooking sauce in Pressure Pot and cook for 3 to 5 minutes or until thickened to desired consistency.

8. Drizzle sauce over lamb steaks and serve.

9. Nutrition info: Calories: 178 Cal, Carbs: 3 g, Fat: 11 g, Protein: 15 g, Fiber: 0.g.

Lamb Chops with Beans & Spinach

Servings: 5

Cooking Time: 32 Minutes

Ingredients:

- 4 (6-ounce) bone-in lamb shoulder chops, trimmed
- 1 small onion, chopped finely
- 2 cups hot water
- 2 cups boiled white beans
- 2 cups fresh spinach leaves, torn
- 2 tablespoons olive oil
- Salt and ground black pepper, as required
- 3 garlic cloves, crushed
- 2 tablespoons fresh lemon juice

Directions:

1. in the Pressure Pot, place oil and press "Sauté". Now add the leg of lamb and sear for about 2 minutes per side or until browned completely.

2. with a slotted spoon, transfer the chops onto a plate.

3. in the pot, add the onion and garlic and cook for about 1-2 minutes.

4. Press "Cancel" and stir in the hot water, salt and black pepper.

5. Arrange the chops in an even layer and submerge into the liquid.

6. Close the lid and place the pressure valve to "Seal" position.

7. Press "Manual" and cook under "High Pressure" for about 20 minutes.

8. Press "Cancel" and allow a "Natural" release for about 10 minutes. Then allow a "Quick" release.

9. Open the lid and transfer lamb chops into a large bowl.

10. with 2 forks shred the meat.

11. Press "Sauté" and cook for about 3-4 minutes.

12. Stir in the lamb meat and beans and cook for about 1-2 minutes or until desired thickness.

13. Press "Cancel" and stir in the spinach until wilted.

14. Stir in lemon juice and serve hot.

15. Nutrition info: Per serving: Calories: 361, Fats: 16.6g, Carbs: 19.3g, Sugar:1.6g, Proteins: 33.5g, Sodium: 181mg

Beef Fajitas

Servings: 4

Cooking Time: 10 Minutes

Ingredients:

• 1-pound steak roast

• 1 medium red onion, peeled and cut into strips

• 1 medium red bell pepper, deseeded and cut into strips

• 1 medium yellow bell pepper, deseeded and cut into strips

• 1 tablespoon taco seasoning

• 2 limes, juiced and zest

• 1/2 cup beef stock

Directions:

1. Cut beef into thin strips and season well with taco seasoning until evenly coated.

2. Plugin Pressure Pot, insert the inner pot, add seasoned beef strips along with remaining onion, peppers and beef stock.

3. Shut the Pressure Pot with its lid, turn the pressure knob to seal the pot, press the „manual" button, then press the „timer" to set the cooking time to 5 minutes

and cook at high pressure, Pressure Pot will take 5 minutes or more for building its inner pressure.

4. When the timer beeps, press „cancel" button and do natural pressure release for 10 minutes and then do quick pressure release until pressure nob drops down.

5. Open the Pressure Pot, add lime juice and zest into beef fajitas and stir until mixed.

6. Serve straight away.

7. Nutrition info: Calories: 123 Cal, Carbs: 9 g, Fat: 3 g, Protein: 14 g, Fiber: 2 g.

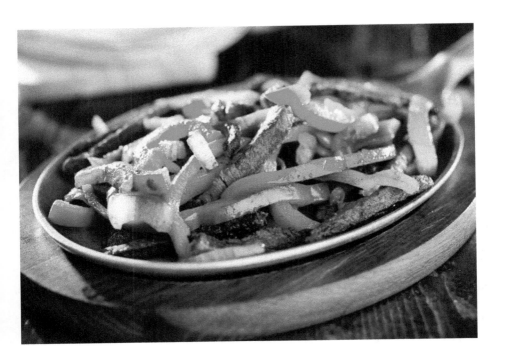

Pork Chops

Servings: 2

Cooking Time: 22 Minutes

Ingredients:

- 2 boneless pork chops, each about 1-inch thick
- 1/2 teaspoon onion powder
- 1 teaspoon salt
- 1 teaspoon ground black pepper
- 2 tablespoons brown sugar
- 1 teaspoon paprika
- 1 tablespoon butter
- 1/2 tablespoon Worcestershire sauce
- 1 cup chicken broth
- 1 teaspoon liquid smoke

Directions:

1. Stir together onion powder, salt, black pepper, sugar, and paprika and rub this mixture on all sides of pork chops until evenly coated.

2. Plugin Pressure Pot, insert the inner pot, press sauté/simmer button, add butter and when it melts, add seasoned pork chops and cook for minutes per side until browned.

3. Press the cancel button, add remaining ingredients and stir until mixed.

4. Shut the Pressure Pot with its lid, turn the pressure knob to seal the pot, press the „manual" button, then press the „timer" to set the cooking time to 7 minutes and cook at high pressure, Pressure Pot will take 5 minutes or more for building its inner pressure.

5. When the timer beeps, press „cancel" button and do natural pressure release for 10 minutes and then do quick pressure release until pressure nob drops down.

6. Open the Pressure Pot, transfer pork chops to a serving plate and let rest for 5 minutes.

7. Drizzle cooking sauce from the Pressure Pot over pork chops and serve straight away.

8. Nutrition info: Calories: 354 Cal, Carbs: 24.5 g, Fat: 16.3 g, Protein: 27.9 g, Fiber: 2 g.

Veal in Milk

Servings: 2

Cooking Time: 35 Minutes

Ingredients:

• 1lb veal steak

• 1lb chopped vegetables

• 2 cups whole milk

• 1tbsp black pepper seasoning mix

Directions:

1. Mix all the ingredients in your Pressure Pot.

2. Cook on Stew for 35 minutes.

3. Release the pressure naturally.

4. Nutrition info: Per serving: Calories: 270;Carbs: 2 ;Sugar: 0 ;Fat: 16 ;Protein: 39 ;GL: 1

Fabada

Servings: 2

Cooking Time: 5 Minutes

Ingredients:

- 0.5lb cubed ham
- 0.5lb black pudding
- 1lb cooked beans
- 1 cup low sodium broth
- 1tbsp spicy seasoning

Directions:

1. Mix all the ingredients in your Pressure Pot.

2. Cook on Stew for 5 minutes. Release the pressure naturally.

3. Nutrition info: Per serving: Calories: 0;Carbs: 20 ;Sugar: 2 ;Fat: 15 ;Protein: 35 ;GL: 9

Pulled Pork

Servings: 2

Cooking Time: 35 Minutes

Ingredients:

• 1.5lb cubed pork

• 1 cup low sodium beef broth

• 0.5 cup low carb BBQ sauce

• 1tbsp spices

Directions:

1. Mix all the ingredients in your Pressure Pot.

2. Cook on Stew for 35 minutes.

3. Release the pressure naturally.

4. Shred the pork.

5. Nutrition info: Per serving: Calories: 340;Carbs: 4 ;Sugar: 1 ;Fat: 22 ;Protein: 4;GL: 1

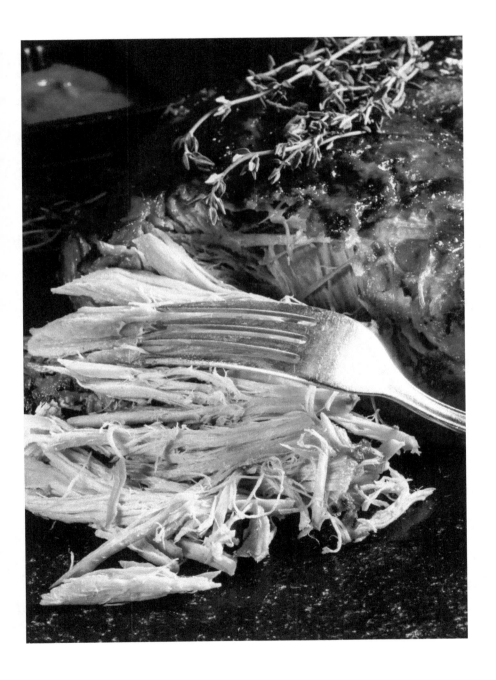

Fruity Pork Loin

Servings: 4

Cooking Time: 40 Minutes

Ingredients:

- 1 1/3 pounds boneless pork tenderloin
- 2 cups apples, cored and chopped
- 2/3 cup fresh cherries, pitted
- ½ cup onion, chopped
- ½ cup fresh apple juice
- Salt and ground black pepper, as required

Directions:

1. in the pot of Pressure Pot, place all ingredients and stir to combine.

2. Close the lid and place the pressure valve to "Seal" position.

3. Press "Meat" and just use the default time of 40 minutes.

4. Press "Cancel" and carefully allow a "Quick" release.

5. Open the lid and transfer the pork onto a cutting board.

6. Cut into desired sized pieces and serve alongside apple mixture.

7. Nutrition info: Per serving: Calories: 255, Fats:4.3g, Carbs: 25,3g, Sugar: 19g, Proteins: 29.2g, Sodium: 339mg

Corned Beef and Cabbage Soup with Barley

Servings: 4

Cooking Time: 20 Minutes

Ingredients:

• 2 tablespoons avocado oil

• 1 small onion, chopped

• 3 celery stalks, chopped

• 3 medium carrots, chopped

• ¼ teaspoon allspice

• 4 cups Chicken Bone Broth, Vegetable Broth, low-sodium store-bought beef broth, or water• 4 cups sliced green cabbage (about ⅓ medium head)

• ¾ cup pearled barley

• 4 ounces cooked corned beef, cut into thin strips or chunks

• Freshly ground black pepper

Directions:

1. Set the electric pressure cooker to the Sauté setting. When the pot is hot, pour in the avocado oil.

2. Sauté the onion, celery, and carrots for 3 to 5 minutes or until the vegetables begin to soften. Stir in

the allspice. Hit Cancel.

3. Stir in the broth, cabbage, and barley.

4. Close and lock the lid of the pressure cooker. Set the valve to sealing.

5. Cook on high pressure for 20 minutes.

6. When the cooking is complete, allow the pressure to release naturally for 10 minutes, then quick release any remaining pressure. Hit Cancel.

7. Once the pin drops, unlock and remove the lid.

8. Stir in the corned beef, season with pepper, and replace the lid. Let the soup sit for about 5 minutes to let the corned beef warm up.

9. Spoon into serving bowls and serve.

10. Nutrition info: Per serving(1¼ CUPS): Calories: 321; Total Fat: 13g; Protein: 11g; Carbohydrates: 42g; Sugars: 7g; Fiber: 11g; Sodium: 412mg

Beef and Rice Stuffed Bell Peppers

Servings: 6

Cooking Time: 30 Minutes

Ingredients:

- 1 ½ cups rice, uncooked
- 4 large green peppers, deseeded and halved
- 1-pound ground beef
- 1 medium white onion, peeled and diced
- 1 medium tomato, diced
- ½ teaspoon salt
- ¼ teaspoon ground black pepper
- 2 cups beef broth
- ¼ cup water
- 1 tablespoon coconut oil

Directions:

1. Plugin Pressure Pot, insert the inner pot, press sauté/simmer button, add oil and when hot, add onion and cook for 5 minutes or until nicely golden brown.

2. Then add beef along with tomatoes, season with salt and black pepper, stir well and cook beef for 5 to 7 minutes or until nicely browned.

3. Add rice, pour in water, stir well and press the cancel

button.

4. Shut the Pressure Pot with its lid, turn the pressure knob to seal the pot, press the „manual" button, then press the „timer" to set the cooking time to 8 minutes and cook at high pressure, Pressure Pot will take 5 minutes or more for building its inner pressure.

5. When the timer beeps, press „cancel" button and do quick pressure release until pressure nob drops down.

6. Open the Pressure Pot, stir well and stuff the rice-beef mixture into a bell pepper.

7. Remove a ¼ cup of the cooking liquid from the Pressure Pot, then arrange stuffed pepper into the pan and shut with lid.

8. Press the „manual" button, then press the „timer" to set the cooking time to 4 minutes and cook at high pressure, Pressure Pot will take 5 minutes or more for building its inner pressure.

9. When the timer beeps, press „cancel" button and do quick pressure release until pressure nob drops down.

10. Serve straight away.

11. Nutrition info: Calories: 306 Cal, Carbs: 9 g, Fat: 14 g, Protein: 33 g, Fiber:3.4 g.

Goat Curry

Servings: 2

Cooking Time: 35 Minutes

Ingredients:

- 1lb diced goat
- 1lb chopped vegetables
- 1 cup chopped tomato
- 1 cup low sodium beef broth
- 1tbsp curry paste

Directions:

1. Mix all the ingredients in your Pressure Pot.

2. Cook on Stew for 35 minutes.

3. Release the pressure naturally.

4. Nutrition info: Per serving: Calories: 390;Carbs: 12 ;Sugar: 5 ;Fat: 19 ;Protein: ;GL: 6

Beef Goulash

Servings: 8

Cooking Time: 45 Minutes

Ingredients:

• 2 pounds beef roast, cut into 1-inch cubes

• 6 medium carrots, peeled and cut into 1-inch pieces

• 1 medium white onion, peeled and cut into 1-inch pieces

• 2 teaspoon salt

• 1/4 cup cornstarch

• 2 tablespoons onion soup mix

• 2 teaspoons paprika

• 2 teaspoons Worcestershire sauce

• 2 cups beef broth

• 2 tablespoon olive oil

• 1/3 cup water

Directions:

1. Cut beef into inch cubes and season with salt.

2. Plugin Pressure Pot, insert the inner pot, press sauté/simmer button, add oil and when hot, add seasoned beef pieces in a single layer and cook for 4 minutes per side or until nicely browned.

3. Cook remaining beef pieces in the same manner, then transfer into a bowl, add onions into the pot and cook for 5 minutes or until sauté.

4. Add carrots, season with paprika and onion soup mix, drizzle with Worcestershire sauce and pour in beef broth.

5. Return beef pieces into the Pressure Pot, stir until just mixed and press the cancel button.

6. Shut the Pressure Pot with its lid, turn the pressure knob toseal the pot, press the „meat/stew" button, then press the „timer" to set the cooking time to 20 minutes and cook at high pressure, Pressure Pot will take 5 minutes or more for building its inner pressure.

7. When the timer beeps, press „cancel" button and do natural pressure release for 10 minutes and then do quick pressure release until pressure nob drops down.

8. Open the Pressure Pot, stir the stew and press the „sauté/simmer" button.

9. Stir together cornstarch and water until combined, add to the Pressure Pot, stir well and cook for 3 minutes or more until cooking sauce is thick to the desired level.

10. Serve straight away.

11. Nutrition info: Calories: 315 Cal, Carbs: 17 g, Fat: 17 g, Protein: 24 g, Fiber: 2 g.

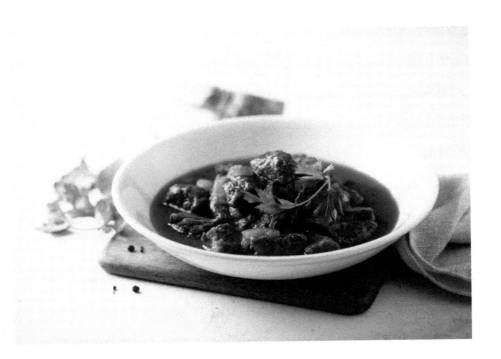

Rosemary Leg of Lamb

Servings: 8

Cooking Time: 55 Minutes

Ingredients:

• 4 pounds boneless leg of lamb

• 2 teaspoons minced garlic

• 2 teaspoons salt

• 1 ½ teaspoon ground black pepper

• 2 tablespoons chopped rosemary

• 2 tablespoons avocado oil, divided

• 2 cups water

Directions:

1. Rinse leg of lamb, pat dry and then season with salt and black pepper.

2. Plugin Pressure Pot, insert the inner pot, press sauté/simmer button, add oil and when hot, add a seasoned leg of lamb and cook for 4 to 5 minutes per side or until nicely browned.

3. Press the cancel button, pour in water, add garlic and rosemary, and insert trivet stand.

4. Place leg of lamb on the stand, shut the Pressure Pot with its lid and turn the pressure knob to seal the pot.

5. Press the „manual" button, then press the „timer" to set the cooking time to 3minutes and cook at high pressure, Pressure Pot will take 5 minutes or more for building its inner pressure.

6. When the timer beeps, press „cancel" button and do natural pressure release for 10 minutes and then do quick pressure release until pressure nob drops down.

7. Open the Pressure Pot, transfer leg of lamb to a cutting board and let cool for 10 minutes.

8. Slice leg of lamb and serve.

9. Nutrition info: Calories: 432 Cal, Carbs:1.02 g, Fat: 25.8 g, Protein: 44.7 g, Fiber: 0.4 g.

Italian Sausage Casserole

Servings: 2

Cooking Time: 5 Minutes

Ingredients:

• 1lb chopped cooked sausages

• 1lb chopped Mediterranean vegetables

• 1 cup low sodium broth

• 1tbsp mixed herbs

Directions:

1. Mix all the ingredients in your Pressure Pot.

2. Cook on Stew for 5 minutes.

3. Release the pressure naturally.

4. Nutrition info: Per serving: Calories: 320;Carbs: 8 ;Sugar: 2 ;Fat: 18 ;Protein: ;GL: 4

Beef Bourguignon Stew

Servings: 6

Cooking Time: 30 Minutes

Ingredients:

- 1 tbsp. butter or olive oil
- 1½ lbs. diced stewing meat
- 4 slices bacon, sliced
- 1 small white onion, diced
- 1 clove garlic, crushed
- 2 stalks celery, sliced
- 8 oz. mushrooms, sliced
- 1 cup low-sodium beef stock
- 1 cup good-quality dry red wine
- 2 tbsp. tomato paste
- 1 bay leaf
- ½ tsp. dried thyme
- ½ tsp. xanthan gum
- ½ tsp. sea salt, or to taste)
- ¼ tsp. freshly ground black pepper
- 1 tbsp. fresh parsley chopped

Directions:

1. Select the "Sauté" function on your Pressure Pot and

sauté the bacon until crispy.

2. Once done, set aside and reserve the bacon grease in the pot.

3. Sear the beef in the Pressure Pot, working in batches to avoid overcrowding the pot and stewing the beef.

4. Discard all but a tablespoon of the drippings from the pot and add a tablespoon of butter or preferred cooking oil.

5. Sauté the onions and celery to the pot, until soft and then add the mushrooms.

6. Stir in the garlic and cook for one minute.

7. Remove all the vegetables and set aside on a side plate.

8. Add xanthan gum to the Pressure Pot, followed by the wine; deglaze the pot thoroughly.

9. Simmer until the wine begins to thicken, and then add the beef broth.

10. Stir in the tomato paste, bay leaf, and thyme, and simmer until the sauce is sufficiently reduced.

11. Return the sautéed vegetables, beef, and bacon to the pot. Stir in the salt and black pepper.

12. Cover and seal the Pressure Pot, making sure the

steam release handle is pointed to "Sealing."

13.Select the "Meat/Stew" function and adjust to cook for 30 minutes.

14. Once done, do a quick pressure release and uncover the stew.

15. Taste and adjust for seasoning, remove and discard the bay leaf and garnish with parsley prior to serving.

16. Nutrition info: Calories 324, Carbs 5g, Fat 18 g, Protein 28g, Potassium (K) 766 mg, Sodium (Na) 124 mg

Balsamic Pork Tenderloin with Raisins

Servings: 4

Cooking Time: 0 Minutes

Ingredients:

• 1½ pounds pork tenderloin (1 tenderloin)

• Kosher salt

• Freshly ground black pepper

• 2 tablespoons avocado oil

• ½ cup unsweetened apple juice or apple cider

• 1 teaspoon herbes de Provence

• ½ teaspoon garlic powder

• 1 tablespoon balsamic vinegar

• ¼ cup unsweetened applesauce or Spiced Pear Applesauce

• ¼ cup golden raisins

Directions:

1. Trim the silver skin from the side of the tenderloin, if necessary. Cut the tenderloin in half crosswise. Season both pieces all over with salt and pepper.

2. Set the electric pressure cooker to the Sauté/More setting. When the pot is hot, pour in the avocado oil.

3. Add the tenderloin pieces to the pot and brown for 5

minutes without turning. Flip and brown the other sides for about minutes. Hit Cancel. Transfer the pork to a plate.

4. Add the apple juice to the pot and scrape up any brown bits from the bottom.

5. Stir in the herbes de Provence, garlic powder, vinegar, applesauce, and raisins. Return the pork to the pot and nestle it into the liquid.

6. Close and lock the lid of the pressure cooker. Set the valve to sealing.

7. Cook on high pressure for 0 minutes (the additional cooking will all occur as the pressure cooker comes to pressure and then naturally releases).

8. When the cooking is complete, hit Cancel. Allow the pressure to release naturally for 15 minutes, then quick release any remaining pressure.

9. Once the pin drops, unlock and remove the lid. Use a meat thermometer to check the internal temperature of the pork. If the pork's temperature is at least 137°F, flip the pork over, replace the lid and let the meat rest for 10 minutes. (The temperature should continue to rise to a safe serving temperature of 145°F.) If the pork's

temperature is less than 137°F, hit Sauté to turn the pressure cooker back on. Cook the pork, turning occasionally, until it reaches a temperature of 137°F. Hit Cancel. Replace the lid and let the meat rest for 10 minutes.

10. Transfer the pork to a cutting board. Thinly slice and serve topped with raisins and sauce.

11. Nutrition info: Per serving: Calories: 300; Total Fat: ; Protein: 36g; Carbohydrates: 13g; Sugars: 10g; Fiber: 1g; Sodium: 186mg.

Spicy Beef Stew with Butternut Squash

Servings: 8

Cooking Time: 30 Minutes

Ingredients:

- 1½ tablespoons smoked paprika
- 2 teaspoons ground cinnamon
- 1½ teaspoons kosher salt
- 1 teaspoon ground ginger
- 1 teaspoon red pepper flakes
- ½ teaspoon freshly ground black pepper
- 2 pounds beef shoulder roast, cut into 1-inch cubes
- 2 tablespoons avocado oil, divided
- 1 cup low-sodium beef or vegetable broth
- 1 medium red onion, cut into wedges
- 8 garlic cloves, minced
- 1 (28-ounce) carton or can no-salt-added diced tomatoes
- 2 pounds butternut squash, peeled and cut into 1-inch pieces
- Chopped fresh cilantro or parsley, for serving

Directions:

1. in a zip-top bag or medium bowl, combine the paprika, cinnamon, salt, ginger, red pepper, and black pepper. Add the beef and toss to coat.

2. Set the electric pressure cooker to the Sauté setting. When the pot is hot, pour in 1 tablespoon of avocado oil.

3. Add half of the beef to the pot and cook, stirring occasionally, for to 5 minutes or until the beef is no longer pink. Transfer it to a plate, then add the remaining 1 tablespoon of avocado oil and brown the remaining beef. Transfer to the plate. Hit Cancel.

4. Stir in the broth and scrape up any brown bits from the bottom of the pot. Return the beef to the pot and add the onion, garlic, tomatoes and their juices, and squash. Stir well.

5. Close and lock lid of pressure cooker. Set the valve to sealing.

6. Cook on high pressure for 30 minutes.

7. When cooking is complete, hit Cancel. Allow the pressure to release naturally for 10 minutes, then quick release any remaining pressure.

8. Unlock and remove lid.

9. Spoon into serving bowls, sprinkle with cilantro or parsley, and serve.

10. Nutrition info: Per serving(1½ CUPS): Calories: 268; Total Fat: ; Protein: 25g; Carbohydrates: 26g; Sugars: 7g; Fiber: 7g; Sodium: 387mg.

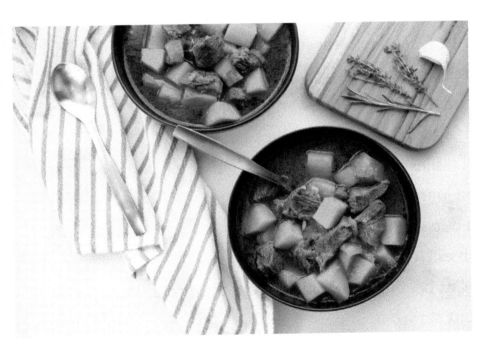

Beef Stroganoff

Servings: 6

Cooking Time: 60 Minutes

Ingredients:

- 2 pounds beef steak
- 1/2 cup flour
- 2 cups sliced mushrooms
- 1 medium white onion, peeled and chopped
- 1 ½ teaspoon minced garlic
- 1/2 teaspoon salt
- 1 tablespoon Worcestershire sauce
- 1/4 teaspoon ground black pepper
- 3 tablespoons olive oil
- 14-ounce beef broth
- 1 cup sour cream

Directions:

1. Cut beef into inch pieces and then coat with ¼ cup flour.

2. Plugin Pressure Pot, insert the inner pot, press sauté/simmer button, add oil and when hot, add coated beef pieces in a single layer and cook for 7 to 10 minutes or until nicely browned.

3. Cook remaining beef pieces in the same manner and then transfer to a bowl.

4. Then add onion and garlic and cook for 3 minutes or until sauté.

5. Add mushrooms, season with salt and black pepper, drizzle with Worcestershire sauce, pour in the broth, then return beef pieces and stir until mixed.

6. Press the cancel button, shut the Pressure Pot with its lid and turn the pressure knob to seal the pot.

7. Press the „manual" button, then press the „timer" to set the cooking time to 30 minutes and cook at high pressure, Pressure Pot will take 5 minutes or more for building its inner pressure.

8. When the timer beeps, press „cancel" button and do natural pressure release for 10 minutes and then do quick pressure release until pressure nob drops down.

9. Open the lid, stir beef stroganoff and if the sauce is too thin, press the „sauté/simmer" button and cook the sauce for 5 minutes or more until sauce is slightly thick.

10. Then press the cancel button, add sour cream into the Pressure Pot and stir until combined.

11. Serve straight away.

12. Nutrition info: Calories: 382.6 Cal, Carbs:13.1 g, Fat: 17.9 g, Protein: 38.2 g, Fiber: 0.9 g.

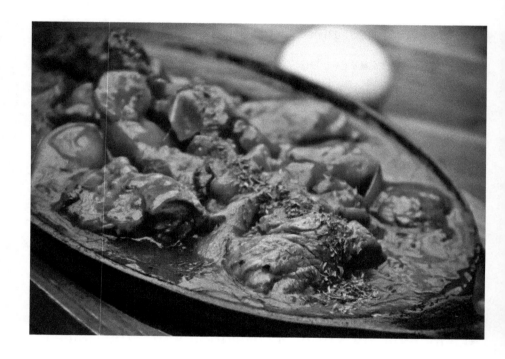

Garlicky Lamb Roast

Servings: 10

Cooking Time: 51 Minutes

Ingredients:

• 1 (3-pound) boneless lamb roast, trimmed

• 3 tablespoons olive oil

• 6 garlic cloves, peeled

• 1 tablespoon dried rosemary

• Salt and ground black pepper, as required

Directions:

1. with a knife, cut small slits all over the lamb roast.

2. Place 1 garlic clove in each cut and press inside.

3. Rub the roast with rosemary and black pepper evenly.

4. in the Pressure Pot, place oil and press "Sauté". Then, add the lamb roast and cook for about 5-6 minutes or until browned completely.

5. Press "Cancel" and transfer the lamb roast onto a plate.

6. Now, arrange a steamer trivet in the Pressure Pot and pour 1 cup of water.

7. Place the lamb roast on top of trivet.

8. Close the lid and place the pressure valve to "Seal" position.

9. Press "Manual" and cook under "High Pressure" for about 45 minutes.

10. Press "Cancel" and allow a "Natural" release.

11. Open the lid and place the lamb roast onto a cutting board for about 5 minutes before slicing.

12. Cut into desired-sized slices and serve.

13. Nutrition info: Per serving: Calories: 293, Fats: 14.2g, Carbs: 0.8g, Sugar: 0g, Proteins: 38.3g, Sodium: 119mg.

DESSERT

Cheesecake

Servings: 8

Cooking Time: 55 Minutes

Ingredients:

For the Filling:

- 16 oz. softened cream cheese
- ¾ cup granulated Swerve sweetener
- ¼ cup heavy whipping cream
- 3 organic eggs
- Zest of 1 small lemon
- 1 tsp. fresh orange zest
- ½ tsp. pure vanilla extract

For the Topping:

- ½ cup sour cream or plain
- 2 tsp. granulated Swerve sweetener

Directions:

1. Wrap baking parchment paper all around the sides of a 6 – 7-inch circular spring form pan.
The paper should be slightly taller than the height of the pan.

2. Lightly grease the bottom of the pan.

3. Tightly wrap aluminum foil all around the bottom of

the pan. Set aside the pan for now.

4. in the bowl of your stand mixer, blend the cream cheese, heavy cream, sweetener, lemon zest, orange zest, and vanilla extract until smooth.

5. Add in the eggs, one at a time, gently mixing until just combined.

6. Be careful not to over mix the eggs, or the cheesecake will be lumpy and not creamy.

7. Pour the cheesecake filling into the prepared pan.

8. Lay a kitchen paper towel over the top of the pan, and gently wrap some aluminum foil. The baking parchment paper will hold the aluminum foil in place.

9. Pour 1½ cups of water into a 6-quart Pressure Pot and place a trivet into the water with the handles facing up.

10. Close and seal the lid, making sure to set the pressure valve to "Sealing".

11. Select the "Manual, High Pressure" function and adjust to cook for 37 minutes.

12. Once the cook cycle ends, allow for a natural pressure release for 18 minutes, and then carefully open the pressure valve and remove the lid.

13. In a small mixing bowl mix together all the ingredients for the topping and set aside for now.

14. Wearing oven mitts, carefully lift out the cheesecake and then remove the foil and kitchen paper from the top.

15. If any condensation has accumulated over the cheesecake, gently dab it off with a kitchen paper towel.

16. While the cheesecake is still warm, spread the topping over it.

17. Place aluminum foil on top the cheesecake and chill for 8 hours, or overnight.

18. Once completely cooled, gently remove the cake from the pan, also removing the outer layer of baking parchment paper, and serve cut into 8 slices.

19. Nutrition info: Calories 268, Carbs 3g, Fat 23.4 g, Protein6.8 g, Potassium (K) 28.8 mg, Sodium (Na) 239.8 mg

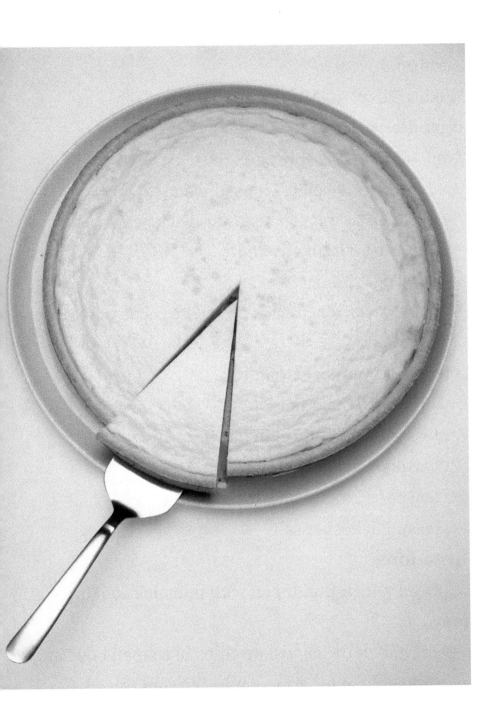

Chipotle Black Bean Brownies

Servings: 8

Cooking Time: 30 Minutes

Ingredients:

- Nonstick cooking spray
- ½ cup dark chocolate chips, divided
- ¾ cup cooked calypso beans or black beans
- ½ cup extra-virgin olive oil
- 2 large eggs
- ¼ cup unsweetened dark chocolate cocoa powder
- ⅓ cup honey
- 1 teaspoon vanilla extract
- ⅓ cup white wheat flour
- ½ teaspoon chipotle chili powder
- ½ teaspoon ground cinnamon
- ½ teaspoon baking powder
- ½ teaspoon kosher salt

Directions:

1. Spray a 7-inch Bundt pan with nonstick cooking spray.

2. Place half of the chocolate chips in a small bowl and microwave them for 30 seconds. Stir and repeat, if

necessary, until the chips have completely melted.

3. in a food processor, blend the beans and oil together. Add the melted chocolate chips, eggs, cocoa powder, honey, and vanilla. Blend until the mixture is smooth.

4. in a large bowl, whisk together the flour, chili powder, cinnamon, baking powder, and salt. Pour the bean mixture from the food processor into the bowl and stir with a wooden spoon until well combined. Stir in the remaining chocolate chips.

5. Pour the batter into the prepared Bundt pan. Cover loosely with foil.

6. Pour 1 cup of water into the electric pressure cooker.

7. Place the Bundt pan onto the wire rack and lower it into the pressure cooker.

8. Close and lock the lid of the pressure cooker. Set the valve to sealing.

9. Cook on high pressure for 30 minutes.

10. When the cooking is complete, hit Cancel and quick release the pressure.

11. Once the pin drops, unlock and remove the lid.

12. Carefully transfer the pan to a cooling rack for about 10 minutes, then invert the cake onto the rack

and let it cool completely.

13. Cut into slices and serve.

14. Nutrition info: Per serving(1 SLICE): Calories: 296; Total Fat: 20g; Protein: 5g; Carbohydrates: 29g; Sugars: 16g; Fiber: 4g; Sodium: 224mg

Chia Vanilla Pudding

Servings: 2

Cooking Time: 10 Minutes

Ingredients:

- 1/4 cup chia seeds
- 2 cups milk
- 4tbsp sweetener
- 1tsp vanilla extract

Directions:

1. Pour the milk into your Pressure Pot.

2. Add the remaining ingredients, stir well.

3. Seal and close the vent.

4. Choose Manual and set to cook 10 minutes.

5. Release the pressure naturally.

6. Nutrition info: Per serving: Calories: 320;Carbs: 11 ;Sugar: ;Fat: 6 ;Protein: 8 ;GL: 7

Chai Pear-Fig Compote

Servings: 4

Cooking Time: 3 Minutes

Ingredients:

- 1 vanilla chai tea bag
- 1 (3-inch) cinnamon stick
- 1 strip lemon peel (about 2-by-½ inches)
- 1½ pounds pears, peeled and chopped (about 3 cups)
- ½ cup chopped dried figs
- 2 tablespoons raisins

Directions:

1. Pour cup of water into the electric pressure cooker and hit Sauté/More. When the water comes to a boil, add the tea bag and cinnamon stick. Hit Cancel. Let the tea steep for 5 minutes, then remove and discard the tea bag.

2. Add the lemon peel, pears, figs, and raisins to the pot.

3. Close and lock the lid of the pressure cooker. Set the valve to sealing.

4. Cook on high pressure for 3 minutes.

5. When the cooking is complete, hit Cancel and quick

release the pressure.

6. Once the pin drops, unlock and remove the lid.

7. Remove the lemon peel and cinnamon stick. Serve warm or cool to room temperature and refrigerate.

8. Nutrition info: Per serving: Calories: 167; Total Fat: 1g; Protein: 2g; Carbohydrates: 44g; Sugars: 29g; Fiber: 9g; Sodium: 4mg.

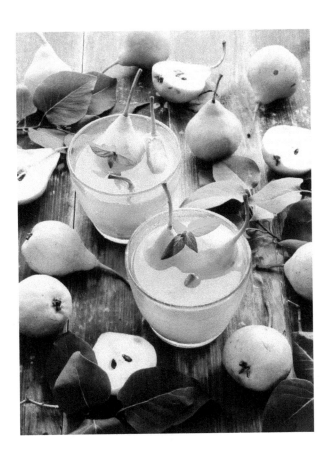

Oatmeal Bites

Servings: 12

Cooking Time: 15 Minutes

Ingredients:

• 1 cup mixed berries, slightly mashed

• 1 cup rolled oats

• 1/2 cup whole wheat flour

• 1/4 teaspoon salt

• 1 tablespoon brown sugar

• 1/2 teaspoon cinnamon

• 1 teaspoon baking powder

• 1/3 cup honey

• 4 eggs

• 1 cup water

Directions:

1. Place oats and flour in a bowl, add salt, cinnamon and baking powder and stir until mixed.

2. Crack eggs in a bowl, add sugar and honey and beat until well combined.

3. Then fold in flour mixture, 4 tablespoons at a time, until incorporated and then fold in berries.

4. Take twelve egg molds, grease them with oil, and

then fill each portion with a scoop of cookie mixture, about 3 tablespoons.

5. Plugin Pressure Pot, insert the inner pot, pour in water, then insert steamer basket and place egg molds on it.

6. Shut the Pressure Pot with its lid, turn the pressure knob to seal the pot, press the „manual" button, then press the „timer" to set the cooking time to 10 minutes and cook at high pressure, Pressure Pot will take 5 minutes or more for building its inner pressure.

7. When the timer beeps, press „cancel" button and do natural pressure release for 10 minutes and then do quick pressure release until pressure nob drops down.

8. Open the Pressure Pot, transfer egg molds to a wire rack to cool oatmeal bites, then take them out and dust with powdered sweetener.

9. Serve straight away.

10. Nutrition info: Calories: 36.7 Cal, Carbs:6.2 g, Fat: 1 g, Protein:1.2 g, Fiber: 0.7 g.

Egg Custard

Servings: 4

Cooking Time: 4 Minutes

Ingredients:

• 1½ cups unsweetened almond milk, divided

• 3 large eggs

• 5 tablespoons Erythritol

• Pinch of salt

Directions:

1. in the pot of Pressure Pot, place cup of almond milk, Erythritol and salt and press "Sauté".

2. Cook for about 3-4 minutes or until Erythritol is dissolved completely, stirring continuously.

3. Press "Cancel" and transfer the almond milk mixture into a bowl.

4. Set aside to cool slightly.

5. in the pot, add remaining almond milk and mix well.

6. in a large glass bowl, add eggs and beat well.

7. Slowly pour the almond t milk mixture, beating continuously until well combined.

8. Through a fine mesh strainer, strain the egg mixture twice.

9. Now, place the egg mixture into 4 (3x1½-inch) ramekins evenly.

10. with a spoon, remove any air bubbles.

11. with 1 foil piece, cover each ramekin tightly.

12. Arrange a steamer trivet in the Pressure Pot and pour 1 cup of water.

13. Place the ramekins on top of trivet.

14. Close the lid and place the pressure valve to "Seal" position.

15. Press "Manual" and cook under "Low Pressure" for about 0 minute.

16. Press "Cancel" and allow a "Natural" release for about 10 minutes. Then allow a "Quick" release.

17. Open the lid and transfer the ramekins onto a wire rack.

18. Remove the foil pieces and set aside to cool slightly.

19. Serve warm.

20. Nutrition info: Per serving: Calories: 69, Fats: 6g, Carbs: 1g, Sugar: 0.3g, Proteins:5.1g, Sodium: 159mg

Bran Porridge

Servings: 2

Cooking Time: 10 Minutes

Ingredients:

- 1/4 cup bran
- 1 cup milk
- 1 cup diabetic applesauce
- 4tbsp sweetener
- 1tsp cinnamon

Directions:

1. Pour the milk into your Pressure Pot.

2. Add the remaining ingredients, stir well.

3. Seal and close the vent.

4. Choose Manual and set to cook 10 minutes.

5. Release the pressure naturally.

6. Nutrition info: Per serving: Calories: 320;Carbs: 12 ;Sugar: 4 ;Fat: 2 ;Protein: 3 ;GL: 4

Chia Pudding with Mango

Servings: 2

Cooking Time: 10 Minutes

Ingredients:

- 1/4 cup chia seeds
- 1 cup orange juice
- 1 cup chopped mango
- 4tbsp sweetener

Directions:

1. Pour the milk into your Pressure Pot.

2. Add the remaining ingredients, stir well.

3. Seal and close the vent.

4. Choose Manual and set to cook 10 minutes.

5. Release the pressure naturally.

6. Nutrition info: Per serving: Calories: 320;Carbs: 12 ;Sugar: 5 ;Fat: ;Protein: 8 ;GL: 7

Brown Rice Pudding

Servings: 6

Cooking Time: 22 Minutes

Ingredients:

- 1 cup long-grain brown rice, rinsed
- 2 cups unsweetened almond milk
- ¼ cup Yacon syrup
- 3 tablespoons almonds, chopped
- ½ teaspoon organic vanilla extract
- ¼ teaspoon ground cinnamon
- Pinch of sea salt

Directions:

1. in the pot of Pressure Pot, place all the ingredients and stir to combine.

2. Close the lid and place the pressure valve to "Seal" position.

3. Press "Manual" and cook under "High Pressure" for about 22 minutes.

4. Press "Cancel" and allow a "Natural" release for about 10 minutes. Then allow a "Quick" release.

5. Open the lid and stir the pudding well.

6. Transfer the pudding into a bowl and set aside to

cool slightly.

7. Serve warm with the topping of almonds.

8. Nutrition info: Per serving: Calories: 163, Fats:3.5g, Carbs: 29g, Sugar:2.5g, Proteins:3.3g, Sodium: 105mg.

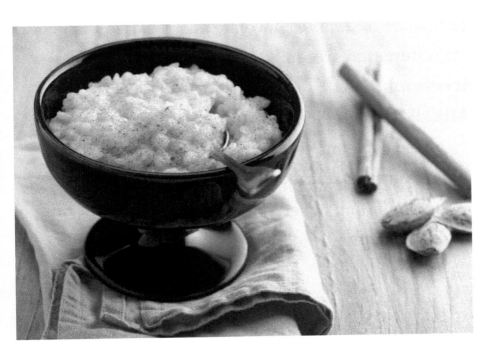

White Chocolate

Servings: 2

Cooking Time: 2 Minutes

Ingredients:

- 4tbsp double cream
- 6tsp powdered sweetener
- 3tsp sugar-free white chocolate mix
- hot water or fat-free milk

Directions:

1. Mix all the ingredients in your Pressure Pot.

2. Seal and cook on Stew for minutes.

3. Depressurize naturally. Stir well and serve.

4. Nutrition info: Per serving: Calories: 105;Carbs: 3 ;Sugar: 1 ;Fat: 12 ;Protein: ;GL: 1

Chili Chocolate

Servings: 2

Cooking Time: 2 Minutes

Ingredients:

- 4tbsp double cream
- 3tsp powdered sweetener
- 3tsp sugar-free pure cocoa
- 1/8tsp chili powder
- hot water or fat-free milk

Directions:

1. Mix all the ingredients in your Pressure Pot.

2. Seal and cook on Stew for minutes.

3. Depressurize naturally.

4. Stir well and serve.

5. Nutrition info: Per serving: Calories: 100;Carbs: 3 ;Sugar: 1 ;Fat: 11 ;Protein: 4 ;GL: 1

Peanut Butter Cookies

Servings: 2

Cooking Time: 5 Minutes

Ingredients:

- 1/3 cup peanut butter
- 1/3 cup dark chocolate chips
- 2tbsp powdered sweetener
- 1tbsp applesauce
- pinch of baking soda

Directions:

1. Mix the sweetener, applesauce, and baking soda together.

2. Add in the peanut butter.

3. Fold in the chocolate chips.

4. Make cookies and lay them out on a heat-proof tray that fits into your Pressure Pot steamer tray.

5. Pour a cup of water into the Pressure Pot.

6. Place the tray in the steamer basket and the basket in the Pressure Pot.

7. Cook on Steam, low pressure, for 20 minutes.

8. Depressurize quickly and serve.

9. Nutrition info: Per serving: Calories: 3;Carbs: 20 ;Sugar: 9 ;Fat: 26 ;Protein: 10 ;GL: 7

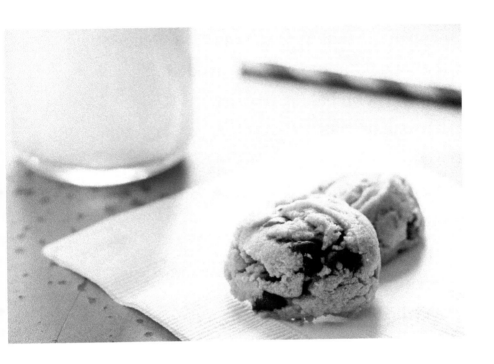

Apple and Cinnamon Cake

Servings: 8

Cooking Time: 65 Minutes

Ingredients:

- 3 large apples, peeled, cored and diced
- 1/2 tablespoon ground cinnamon
- ¾ cup and 2 tablespoons swerve sweetener
- 1 1/2 cups flour and more as needed
- 1/2 tablespoon baking powder
- 1/2 teaspoon salt
- 1/2 cup olive oil
- 1 teaspoon vanilla extract, unsweetened
- 2 eggs
- 1 cup water

Directions:

1. Place diced apples in a bowl, add cinnamon and 2 tablespoons sweetener and toss until evenly coated, set aside until required.

2. Place flour in a large bowl, add salt and baking powder and stir until mixed.

3. Crack eggs in another bowl, add vanilla, oil and remaining sugar and beat until well combined.

4. Then stir in flour mixture, tablespoons at a time, until incorporated and then pour half of this mixture into a greased 7-inch cake pan.

5. Spread half of the apples on the batter in a cake pan, then pour remaining batter on the apple pieces and scatter remaining apples on top along with any juices.

6. Plugin Pressure Pot, insert the inner pot, pour in water, and insert a steamer basket.

7. Cover cake pan with aluminum foil, then place it on the steamer basket, shut the Pressure Pot with its lid and turn the pressure knob to seal the pot.

8. Press the „manual" button, then press the „timer" to set the cooking time to 60 minutes and cook at high pressure, Pressure Pot will take 5 minutes or more for building its inner pressure.

9. When the timer beeps, press „cancel" button and do quick pressure release until pressure nob drops down.

10. Open the Pressure Pot, take out the cake pan, uncover it, and let the cake cool on wire rack.

11. Slice the cake and serve.

12. Nutrition info: Calories: 275 Cal, Carbs: 35 g, Fat: 14 g, Protein: 2 g, Fiber: 1 g.

Pumpkin Custard

Servings: 6

Cooking Time: 20 Minutes

Ingredients:

- 15 oz. can pumpkin puree
- ½ cup coconut milk
- ⅔ cup real maple syrup
- 1 egg
- ½ tsp. pumpkin pie spice
- Cooking oil spray

Directions:

1. Spray a 6-inch cake pan with cooking oil spray.

2. Place a metal trivet into a 6-quart Pressure Pot, along with cups of water.

3. in a medium-sized mixing bowl, combine the pumpkin puree, maple syrup, coconut milk, egg, and pumpkin pie spice. Stir well.

4. Pour the pudding mixture into the cake pan and gently place the pan into the Pressure Pot.

5. Lock the lid and select the „Manual, High Pressure" button. Cook for 20 minutes.

6. Once done, let the naturally release the pressure or

use the quick-release method.

7. Gently remove the cake pan from the Pressure Pot.

8. Using a serving spoon, divide the pudding between six serving bowls.

9. Serve hot or at room temperature.

10. Nutrition info: Calories 165, Carbs 29.9g, Fat 5g, Protein2.2 g, Potassium (K) 305.7 mg, Sodium (Na) 22.1 mg

Pecan Pie Cheesecake

Servings: 10

Cooking Time: 35 Minutes

Ingredients:

For the Crust:

- ¾ cup almond flour
- 2 tbsps. melted butter
- 2 tbsps. powdered Swerve sweetener
- ⅛ tsp. salt

For the Pecan Pie Filling:

- ¼ cup butter
- ½ cup chopped pecans
- 1 beaten egg
- ⅓ cup powdered Swerve
- 2 tbsps. heavy whipping cream
- 1 tsp. molasses
- 1 tsp. pure caramel extract
- ¼ tsp. sea salt

For the Cheesecake Filling:

- 12 oz. softened cream cheese
- 1 beaten egg
- ¼ cup heavy whipping cream

- 5 tbsps. powdered Swerve sweetener
- ½ tsp. pure vanilla extract

For the Cheesecake Topping:

- 2½ tbsps. powdered Swerve
- 2 tbsps. butter
- ½ tsp. molasses
- 1 tbsp. heavy whipping cream
- ½ tsp. pure caramel extract
- Whole toasted pecans

Directions:

1. To make the Crust:

2. Whisk the almond flour, powdered sweetener, and salt in a medium-sized mixing bowl.

3. Stir in the melted butter until the mixture comes together.

4. Press into the bottom and halfway up the sides of a 7-inch circular spring form pan.

5. Freeze as you make the rest of the recipe.

6. To make the Pie Filling:

7. in a small saucepan melt the butter over low heat.

8. Add the molasses and powdered sweetener, and whisk until combined.

9. Stir in the caramel or vanilla extract and heavy whipping cream, and then stirring, add the egg. The mixture will thicken as it continues to cook over low heat.

10. Immediately remove the filling from heat and stir in the chopped pecans and salt.

11. Spread the mixture over the bottom of the frozen crust and set aside.

12. To make the Cheesecake Filling:

13. Whisk together the cream cheese until softened and smooth, and then beat in the powdered sweetener.

14. Beat in the whipping cream, egg, and vanilla extract.

15. Pour this cheesecake filling over the pecan pie filling and spread to the edges of the pan.

16. To bake the Cheesecake:

17. Tightly wrap the bottom of the circular spring form pan with aluminum foil.

18. Place a large piece of kitchen paper over the top of the spring form pan, making sure it does not touch the cheesecake, and then wrap aluminum foil over the top as well.

19. Place the pan on a steam wire rack inside your Pressure Pot and pour a cup of water into the bottom of the pot.

20. Carefully lower the wrapped cake pan onto the steamer rack.

21.Close and seal the lid, making sure the pressure release valve is set to "Sealing" and then cook on the "Manual, High Pressure" setting for 30 minutes.

22. Once the baking is complete, allow for a natural pressure release.

23. Carefully remove the cheesecake and cool to room temperature, and then chill for 3-4 hours, or even overnight, before topping and serving.

24. To make the Topping:

25. in a small saucepan melt the butter over low heat.

26. Add the powdered sweetener and molasses and whisk until well combined.

27. Stir in the caramel or vanilla extract and heavy whipping cream.

28. Drizzle this topping over the chilled cheesecake and garnish with toasted whole pecans.

29. Nutrition info: Calories 340, Carbs4.97g, Fat 31.03

g, Protein5.89g, Potassium (K) 204.4 mg, Sodium (Na) 252.0 mg

Chocolate Cheesecake

Servings: 8

Cooking Time: 25 Minutes

Ingredients:

- For the Crust:
- ¼ cup coconut flour
- ¼ cup almond flour
- 2½ tbsps. unsweetened cocoa powder
- 2 tbsps. butter melted
- 1½ tbsps. low-carb sweetener
- For the Filling:
- ¼ cup sour cream
- ¾ cup heavy cream
- ⅓ cup unsweetened cocoa powder
- 16 oz. cream cheese, room temperature
- ½ tsp. monk fruit powder
- ½ tsp. stevia concentrated powder
- 2 large egg yolks
- 1 large egg
- 6 oz. baking chocolate melted
- 1 tsp. pure vanilla extract

Directions:

1. Crust:

2. Line bottom of a 7-inch spring form pan with baking parchment paper cut to fir the pan.

3. Combine all the dry crust ingredients and then stir in melted butter.

4. Using clean fingers, press the crust into the bottom of prepared pan and chill.

5. Filling:

6. Using an electric mixer blend the cream cheese, cocoa powder, and sweeteners. and cocoa powder.

7. Blend in the large egg, and then the egg yolks.

8. Add the heavy cream, sour cream, melted chocolate, and pure vanilla extract.

9. Scrape the sides of the bowl to incorporate the ingredients as needed.

10. Pour the cream cheese mixture on to the crust in the pan. Smooth the top of the filling using a rubber spatula.

11. Place a wire steamer rack in the Pressure Pot, and then add in 1½ cups of water.

12. Make an aluminum foil sling and place over the

steamer rack making sure the ends are long enough to extend to the top of the Pressure Pot.

13. Place the cheesecake pan over the sling and cover loosely with aluminum foil to prevent any condensation from dripping on top.

14. Fold the tops of the sling loosely over the cheesecake.

15.Cover the Pressure Pot and cook at „Manual, High Pressure" for 20 minutes.

16. When the time is up, allow the pot to release the pressure naturally for 15 minutes.

17. Open the lid and gently lift the cheesecake out and set onto a cooling rack.

18. Allow to cool for 1 hour and then chill for a 2 – 3 hours before removing the side of the pan.

19. For the best results, the cheesecake should sit overnight in the refrigerator.

20. Serve at room temperature for a softer texture.

21. Nutrition info: Calories 413, Carbs 1g, Fat 38 g, Protein 8 g, Potassium (K) 319 mg, Sodium (Na) 56 mg

Rich Wild Rice Pudding

Servings: 2

Cooking Time: 10 Minutes

Ingredients:

- 1/4 cup dry wild rice
- 1 cup milk
- 6 squares 90% dark chocolate
- 4tbsp sweetener
- 1tsp mixed spice

Directions:

1. Pour the milk into your Pressure Pot.

2. Add the remaining ingredients, stir well.

3. Seal and close the vent.

4. Choose Manual and set to cook 10 minutes.

5. Release the pressure naturally.

6. Nutrition info: Per serving: Calories: 320;Carbs: 14 ;Sugar: 2 ;Fat: 2 ;Protein: 3 ;GL: 5

Low Carb Custard

Servings: 2

Cooking Time: 20 Minutes

Ingredients:

• 2 eggs

• 2oz cream cheese

• 1.5tbsp powdered sweetener

• 1.5tsp caramel sauce

• 1 cup water

Directions:

1. Blend the ingredients together.

2. Pour into a heat-proof bowl that fits into your Pressure Pot.

3. Pour a cup of water into the Pressure Pot.

4. Place the bowl in the steamer basket and the basket in the Pressure Pot.

5. Cook on Steam, low pressure, for 20 minutes.

6. Depressurize quickly and serve.

7. Nutrition info: Per serving: Calories: 2;Carbs:1.5 ;Sugar: 0 ;Fat: 27 ;Protein: 9 ;GL: 1

Glazed Apples

Servings: 6

Cooking Time: 2 Minutes

Ingredients:

• 3 gala apples, peeled, core and sliced

• 1 teaspoon Yacon syrup

• ¼ cup water

• 1 teaspoon ground cinnamon

Directions:

1. in the pot of Pressure Pot, place all the ingredients and mix well.

2. Close the lid and place the pressure valve to "Seal" position.

3. Press "Manual" and cook under "High Pressure" for about 2 minutes.

4. Press "Cancel" and carefully allow a "Quick" release.

5. Open the lid and serve immediately.

6. Nutrition info: Per serving: Calories: 37, Fats: 0.3g, Carbs:8., Sugar:7.2g, Proteins: 0.1g, Sodium: 0mg

Strawberry Compote

Servings: 4

Cooking Time: 4 Minutes

Ingredients:

- 1 pound fresh strawberries, hulled, sliced and divided
- ¼ cup Yacon syrup
- 1 teaspoon fresh lemon zest, grated
- 2 tablespoons fresh lemon juice
- 1 teaspoon organic vanilla extract

Directions:

1. in the pot of Pressure Pot, place ¾ pound of strawberries and remaining ingredients and stir to combine.

2. Close the lid and place the pressure valve to "Seal" position.

3. Press "Manual" and cook under "High Pressure" for about 1 minute.

4. Press "Cancel" and allow a "Natural" release for about 10 minutes. Then allow a "Quick" release.

5. Open the lid and press "Sauté".

6. Cook for about 3 minutes, crushing the strawberries slightly with the back of a wooden spoon.

7. Stir in remaining strawberries and Press "Cancel".

8. Transfer compote into a bowl and set aside in room temperature to cool completely.

9. Refrigerate before serving.

10. Nutrition info: Per serving: Calories: 66, Fats: 0.4g, Carbs: 15g, Sugar:9.4g, Proteins: 0.8g, Sodium: 9mg.

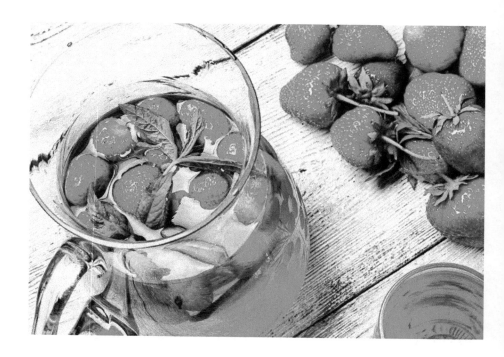

Brownies

Servings: 16

Cooking Time: 55 Minutes

Ingredients:

- 3/4 cup whole wheat flour
- 1/2 teaspoon salt
- 1/2 teaspoon baking powder
- 1/2 cup cocoa powder, unsweetened
- 1 cup swerve sweetener
- 1 cup chocolate chips, unsweetened
- 1 teaspoon vanilla extract, unsweetened
- 1/2 cup butter, soften
- 2 eggs
- 1 ½ cup water

Directions:

1. Place butter in a bowl, cream with a beater, then beat in sweetener until combined and beat in eggs and vanilla until incorporated.

2. Place flour in a bowl, add salt, baking powder, cocoa powder and stir until combined.

3. Stir the flour mixture into the egg mixture, 2 tablespoons at a time, until incorporated and then fold

in chocolate chips until combined.

4. Take a 7 by 3 push pan or pan that fits into the Pressure Pot, grease it with oil, then spoon in prepared batter, smooth the top and cover with aluminum foil.

5. Plugin Pressure Pot, insert the inner pot, pour in water, insert trivet stand and place brownie pan on it.

6. Shut the Pressure Pot with its lid, turn the pressure knob to seal the pot, press the „manual" button, then press the „timer" to set the cooking time to 50 minutes and cook at high pressure, Pressure Pot will take 5 minutes or more for building its inner pressure.

7. When the timer beeps, press „cancel" button and do natural pressure release for 10 minutes and then do quick pressure release until pressure nob drops down.

8. Open the Pressure Pot, remove the pan, uncover it and let brownies cool in pan on wire rack.

9. Cut brownies into squares and serve.

10. Nutrition info: Calories: 200 Cal, Carbs: 24 g, Fat: 11 g, Protein: 2 g, Fiber: 1 g.

Almond Pudding

Servings: 2

Cooking Time: 2 Minutes

Ingredients:

- 2 cups unsweetened almond milk
- ¾-1 cup almond meal
- 1 tablespoon Erythritol
- Pinch of saffron strands, crushed
- 1/8 teaspoon ground cardamom

Directions:

1. In the pot of Pressure Pot, place all ingredients and stir to combine.
2. Close the lid and place the pressure valve to "Seal" position.
3. Press "Manual" and cook under "High Pressure" for about 2 minutes.
4. Press "Cancel" and allow a "Natural" release.
5. Open the lid and transfer the pudding into a bowl.
6. Remove the foil pieces and set aside to cool slightly.
7. Serve warm.
8. Nutrition info: Per serving: Calories: 247, Fats:

21.3g, Carbs:9., Sugar:1.5g, Proteins:8.6g, Sodium: 180mg.

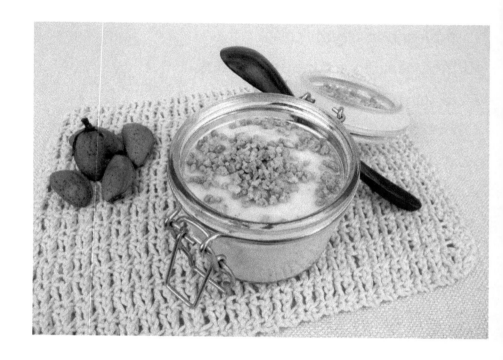

Apple Crisp

Servings: 4

Cooking Time: 10 Minutes

Ingredients:

- 4 cups apples, cored and chopped
- 2/3 cup rolled oats
- 1/3 cup almond flour
- 9 pecans, chopped
- 2 tablespoons plus 2 teaspoons Yacon syrup, divided
- 4 teaspoon olive oil
- 1 teaspoon fresh lemon juice
- ½ teaspoon fresh lemon zest, grated
- ¾ teaspoon ground cinnamon, divided
- Pinch of salt

Directions:

1. For filling: in a bowl, add the apple pieces, 2 teaspoons of Yacon syrup, lemon zest, lemon juice and ½ teaspoon of cinnamon and toss to coat well. Set aside.

2. For topping: in another bowl, add the oats, pecans, almond flour, oil, tablespoon of Yacon syrup, ¼ teaspoon of cinnamon and salt and mix well.

3. Divide the apple mixture into 4 ramekins evenly and top with oats mixture.

4. Arrange a steamer trivet in the Pressure Pot and pour 1 cup of water.

5. Place the ramekins on top of trivet.

6. Close the lid and place the pressure valve to "Seal" position.

7. Press "Manual" and cook under "High Pressure" for about minutes.

8. Meanwhile, preheat the oven to broiler.

9. Press "Cancel" and carefully allow a "Quick" release.

10. Open the lid and arrange the ramekins onto a baking sheet in a square.

11. Broil for about 2-3 minutes or until top just starts to brown.

12. Remove from oven and place the ramekins onto a wire rack to cool for about 10 minutes before serving.

Nutrition info: Per serving: Calories: 336, Fats: 16.5g, Carbs: 46.2g, Sugar: 25g, Proteins:3.3g, Sodium: 45mg.

Poached Spiced Pears

Servings: 4

Cooking Time: 12 Minutes

Ingredients:

• 4 medium pears, peeled

• 1 lemon, juiced

• 1-star anise

• 1 stick of cinnamon

• 3 cups white grape juice

• 3½ cups water

Directions:

1. Plugin Pressure Pot, insert the inner pot, add all the ingredients except for pears and stir until just mixed.

2. Then add pears, shut the Pressure Pot with its lid and turn the pressure knob to seal the pot.

3. Press the „manual" button, then press the „timer" to set the cooking time to 8 minutes and cook at high pressure, Pressure Pot will take 5 minutes or more for building its inner pressure.

4. When the timer beeps, press „cancel" button and do natural pressure release for 10 minutes and then do quick pressure release until pressure nob drops down.

5. Open the Pressure Pot, transfer pears to serving plates and drizzle with cooking liquid.

6. Serve straight away.

7. Nutrition info: Calories: 136 Cal, Carbs: 22 g, Fat: 0.2 g, Protein: 0.6 g, Fiber: 9 g.

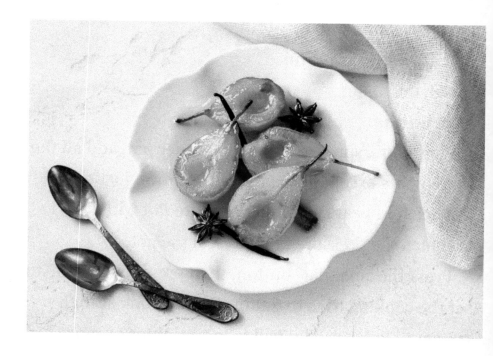

Carrot Cake

Servings: 6

Cooking Time: 55 Minutes

Ingredients:

- For Cake:
- 2 cups grated carrots
- 1 banana, mashed
- 1 1 /2 cup whole-meal flour
- ¼ cup sultanas
- 2 teaspoons mixed spice
- 1 teaspoon baking powder
- 3 tablespoons swerve sweetener
- ¼ cup rapeseed oil
- 3 eggs, slightly beaten
- 1 cup water
- For Frosting:
- 1 orange, zested
- 1 ¼ cup cream cheese, fat-free
- 1 tablespoon swerve sweetener

Directions:

1. Place flour in a bowl, add mixed spice and baking powder and stir until mixed.

2. Crack eggs in another bowl, add banana and beat the mixture until well combined.

3. Then beat in sweetener and oil until incorporated and then stir in flour mixture, 4 tablespoons at a time, until incorporated and smooth batter comes together.

4. Fold carrots and sultanas into the cake batter, then spoon the mixture into a greased cake pan and cover with aluminum foil.

5. Plugin Pressure Pot, insert the inner pot, pour in water, then insert trivet stand and place the cake pan on it.

6. Shut the Pressure Pot with its lid, turn the pressure knob to seal the pot, press the „steam" button, then press the „timer" to set the cooking time to 50 minutes and cook at high pressure, Pressure Pot will take 5 minutes or more for building its inner pressure.

7. Meanwhile, prepare frosting and for this, beat together orange zest, cream cheese and swerve sweetener until smooth and chill it in the refrigerator until required.

8. When the timer beeps, press „cancel" button and do quick pressure release until pressure nob drops down.

9. Open the Pressure Pot, take out the cake, uncover it, and let the cake cool on wire rack.

10. Then transfer cake to a plate, spread prepared cream cheese frosting on tip and slice to serve.

11. Nutrition info: Calories: 139 Cal, Carbs: 17.3 g, Fat: 5 g, Protein:5.8 g, Fiber:2.6 g.

Chocolate Chip Banana Cake

Servings: 8

Cooking Time: 25 Minutes

Ingredients:

• Nonstick cooking spray

• 3 ripe bananas

• ½ cup buttermilk

• 3 tablespoons honey

• 1 teaspoon vanilla extract

• 2 large eggs, lightly beaten

• 3 tablespoons extra-virgin olive oil

• 1½ cups whole wheat pastry flour

• ⅛ teaspoon ground nutmeg

• 1 teaspoon ground cinnamon

• ¼ teaspoon salt

• 1 teaspoon baking soda

• ⅓ cup dark chocolate chips

Directions:

1. Spray a 7-inch Bundt pan with nonstick cooking spray.

2. in a large bowl, mash the bananas. Add the buttermilk, honey, vanilla, eggs, and olive oil, and mix

well.

3. In a medium bowl, whisk together the flour, nutmeg, cinnamon, salt, and baking soda.

4. Add the flour mixture to the banana mixture and mix well. Stir in the chocolate chips. Pour the batter into the prepared Bundt pan. Cover the pan with foil.

5. Pour 1 cup of water into the electric pressure cooker. Place the pan on the wire rack and lower it into the pressure cooker.

6. Close and lock the lid of the pressure cooker. Set the valve to sealing.

7. Cook on high pressure for 25 minutes.

8. When the cooking is complete, hit Cancel and quick release the pressure.

9. Once the pin drops, unlock and remove the lid.

10. Carefully transfer the pan to a cooling rack, uncover, and let it cool for minutes.

11. Invert the cake onto the rack and let it cool for about an hour.

12. Slice and serve the cake.

13. Nutrition info: Per serving(1 SLICE): Calories: 261;

Total Fat: 11g; Protein: 6g; Carbohydrates: 39g; Sugars: 16g; Fiber: 4g; Sodium: 239mg.

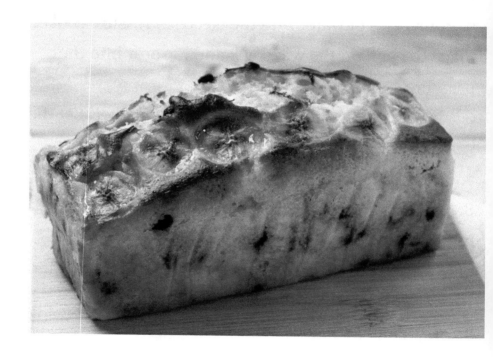

Spiced Pear Applesauce

Servings: 3½ Cups

Cooking Time: 5 Minutes

Ingredients:

• 2 pounds apples, peeled, cored, and sliced

• 1 pound pears, peeled, cored, and sliced

• 2 teaspoons apple pie spice or cinnamon

• Pinch kosher salt

• Juice of ½ small lemon

Directions:

1. in the electric pressure cooker, combine the apples, pears, apple pie spice, salt, lemon juice, and ¼ cup of water.

2. Close and lock the lid of the pressure cooker. Set the valve to sealing.

3. Cook on high pressure for 5 minutes.

4. When the cooking is complete, hit Cancel and let the pressure release naturally.

5. Once the pin drops, unlock and remove the lid.

6. Mash the apples and pears with a potato masher to the consistency you like.

7. Serve warm, or cool to room temperature and

refrigerate.

8. Nutrition info: Per serving(½ CUP): Calories: 10 Total Fat: 1g; Protein: 1g; Carbohydrates: 29g; Sugars: 20g; Fiber: 6g; Sodium: 15mg

Lightning Source UK Ltd.
Milton Keynes UK
UKHW021443200721
387459UK00004B/36

9 781803 424149